Reasons or Results

Life-long Fat-loss System©

Burn Fat Faster
Than You Imagined Possible...

up to 45 pounds in 8 weeks!

*And learn the secrets
to keep it off permanently.*

**Free 1-hour consultation
with the author with purchase of this book.**

by

Sovereign M. Valentine,
Fat-loss Specialist
CFT, Cft, SPN, SSC, GFI, YFI, SFI, CMCht, Reiki Master, CERT, LFR

20+ years professional experience.

https://sovereign-valentine.mykajabi.com

About The Author

Sovereign Valentine has invested the last four decades studying, experimenting and applying general fitness principles, as well as perfecting the fat-loss principles contained herein. He has 37 years experimenting and applying nutrition and close to 30 years as a personal trainer and health professional.

After witnessing first-hand, the affects of poor lifestyle choices within his family and breaking free of the junk food and sugar addiction behaviors himself, he has been refining and practicing what he preaches for the last three decades. During that time, Sov personally invested tens-of-thousands of dollars experimenting to find out what products and ideas are hoaxes and which ones are actually effective and work with those who commit to applying them.

Through an intensive and extensive trial-and-error process and by consistently doing what was purported to work he found what really *does* work. He then goes about documenting the results with each client.

In Sov's words, *"There is no longer a mystery to healthy, sustainable fat-loss. The science and art have been figured out...there aren't any exceptions...it simply comes down to doing the correct things at the correct times and refining as you go. If you think you're an exception, you're not!"*

Sovereign began his formal training as a health care professional with a sincere desire to work with athletes. From a combination of formal training and experimenting, he developed a system that absolutely works.

Sovereign says, *"If you aren't burning between 12 to 20 pounds of fat per month, something is off. A properly designed and executed exercise and nutrition program will facilitate these numbers, (as well as improve overall health) unless you aren't following-through correctly. Without a way to know if you're on track, weeks could go by and you wouldn't even know if you're off track."*

In 1992, he became a Licensed Massage Therapist in Washington State. In 1994 he began doing small, informal nutrition presentations so that others could experience the profound impact that real nutrition has on the body. In 1996, he became a foot and hand reflexologist as well as an energetic healing master. In 1997, he became a certified hypno-therapist. In 1998, he began training others in hypnotherapy and in 1999 he became the first person ever at The Gabriel Institute to be certified as a Master Clinical Hypnotherapist. He went on to become certified in Fitness Training, Fitness Therapy, Sports Conditioning, Endurance Conditioning, a Specialist in Performance Nutrition as well as a Youth Conditioning Specialist, Golf Fitness Instructor, Senior Fitness Specialist and Community Emergency Response Team Member and Licensed Emergency First Responder.

Sovereign's thorough understanding of the systems of the body and how they relate to one another is reflected in his ability to fine-tune his client's training and nutritional regimes for extra-ordinary *Results!* His published works include:

• *Reasons or Results Performance Nutrition Training.*

• *Weighting To Wait; The Emotions of Permanent Fat-loss.*

• *Be Your Own Personal Trainer.*

• *If I were her Trainer.*

• *50-ish Reasons: Why actively and purposely withholding the B.N.B.B.s from your boy is a really bad idea*

Foreword

The fitness, nutrition and weight loss industries have been evolving over the last hundred-years, but especially so in the last forty-years, as being overweight and obese, as well as diabetes and all the other *dis*-eases that accompany being overweight have increased to epidemic proportions.

Generally speaking, the amount of available health and fitness information is simply crazy. But accurate, science-based information which produces healthy, consistent results that can be maintained over the long haul is simple in nature, but challenging to isolate. Much of what's out there is simply about spewing marketing and advertising solutions for some problem symptoms (being overweight and in pain) and then saying, *"Here, take this and all your problems will be solved."*

The truth of the matter, after applying this kind of information for more than three decades, on both myself and with my clients, is that there truly are good nutritional products that make weight loss easier, faster and with less effort, but they are few and far between and the general public simply can't tell a good product from an ineffective one. That's a part of what I do...*assure quality and success through health improvement to prevent and reduce suffering.*

In the United States right now, the right people are doing the right research to help you get real *Results!* At the same time, most food products and dietary supplements for sale really have little nutrition at all, resulting in a lot of missed opportunities by people who could have gotten better *Results!* but to this day don't know why they don't know.

When you hear the words 'fad diet', what they're talking about is either a good program that people picked away at until there wasn't any relevant nutritional content left (requires lifestyle change). Or, the program promised weight loss, fitness and athletic results without exercise and nutritional density to begin with. With any health and fitness program, if the amount of nutritional density isn't increased and isn't provided to your body consistently, you simply won't stick with it since there's no pay off to your chemistry of the brain and body, without additional, consistent nutrition-density.

Secondly, any program that suggests you can burn off all the fat and gain health in all ways, but is without some kind of resistance training [and] cardiovascular/aerobic exercise, its a pipe dream designed to appeal to people who feel frustrated, depressed, sad, defeated and helpless...feeling like they can't do it anymore...empty promises...*hype*...-a bait-and-switch.

The true secret is finding a trainer who has your overall health in mind (not just short-term results) [your health should be improving and you should be feeling better as time goes on] and a trainer who has enough expertise to not only design an amazingly effective program, but one who knows how to adjust the program to you for most effectiveness. Most trainers can design a program, but many don't know how to adjust the program if progress slows down or progress hits a plateau (accountability for both the client and the trainer). This is the second part of what I do.

One of the things that makes me so effective as a trainer is that I've been doing this so long, that when a client isn't getting results, I can narrow it down to whether it has something with the actual workouts, the thoughts & attitudes of the client, the nutritional aspect or if it's in the application of the program during the hours when the client isn't with me.

There simply aren't any mysteries to healthy, sustainable fat-loss to me anymore. A majority of trainers don't stick with the industry long enough to find out what *they didn't know*...I have.

This book lays it out there in simple, concise form and states the basics from many angles and view points, so there's no question what has to happen as you progress through this book.

When you apply these tactics in the way I show you here, you and those who know you will be blown away by the *Results!* you are getting. This book is for people who want the results that speak for themselves...anyone can get some results in the short-run...every 'die-it' will produce some kind of results in the short-run, but most quick, fitness programs erode the physical health after leaving you malnourished, tired, exhausted and depleted...resulting in decreased health and vitality.

Any health-building fitness program should leave you feeling lighter, clearer, relaxed, rejuvenated and more vital than when you started, as well as free of all cravings and any attraction to junk food.

Apply this information and you will be so glad you did...*I promise.*

Read this book now; start getting better today and I look forward to seeing and hearing how good you feel about the *Results!* you are getting!

Once you've read the material, if you're the type to recognize what is real and not just the next fad and if you're willing to commit and follow through until the end, *I'll be there with you every step of the way.*

Acknowledgments

I have not attempted to cite in the text all the authorities and sources in the preparation of this book. To do so would require more space than is available, in order to effectively serve you who apply this information. The list would include departments of the federal government, libraries, industrial institutions, web sources and many individuals as well as my personal experiences and those of my clients since the late 1980's.

Inspiration was contributed by all those before me who succeeded as best they could with the information they had at the time, as well as all those after me who will improve upon this information to make the lives of others better. This book is a culmination of hundreds of books I read, thousands of hours of experimentation and thousands of hours of observing the why, how and where of my own and others' successes and failures.

A Word From The Author

Do it!

This is a *do it* book…read it, learn it…*do it.* If you don't apply it as instructed you'll miss out. Reading this book provides the information but is not the same as doing.

If you need help, contact me!

I work to make a living, but I live to see you get *Results!*

Sovereign Michael Valentine,

April 2018.

Disclaimer

This book is designed to provide information about the subject matter covered. It is produced and sold with the understanding that the publisher and author are not engaged in rendering neither medical diagnosis nor treatment. If you need medical help, go get it. It is not the purpose of this manual to reprint all the information that is otherwise available from other health professionals, but to complement, amplify and supplement other texts. *Reasons or Results! Life-long Fat-loss Program* is neither a cure-all nor a quick-fix for poor lifestyle habits or tendencies. Anyone who commits to personal accountability for their health must expect to re-direct some time, energy and money without any guarantee for specific benefits within a fixed time frame. *Nature works at her own pace.*

Every effort has been made to make this book as complete and accurate as possible. However, there may be mistakes both typographical and in content. Therefore, this book should be used as a general guide and not as the ultimate source of health and nutritional information. Your uniqueness will shine through as you succeed.

The purpose of this book is to educate and inform. The very best results will come from participation. Neither the publisher nor the author shall have responsibility to any person or entity with respect to any loss or damage caused by or alleged to be caused directly or indirectly by the information contained in this book.

This book is not meant to replace the advice or treatments prescribed by your doctor, but rather to accompany your physician's advice. It is not meant to encourage medical treatment of illness or disease or any medical problem by the layperson. It is meant to inform you and open you to health choices that are available to those who seek a broader knowledge. Any application of the ideas set forth in this book is at the applicant's discretion and sole risk. If you are under a doctor's care for any condition, she or he can advise you *about information she or he is familiar with and which she or he has personally experienced.*

The information in this book is neither diagnostic nor prescriptive. It is informational only. The data and information contained herein are based upon information from various peer-reviewed, published and unpublished sources and merely represent training, experience, health and nutrition literature and practices summarized.

Neither the publisher nor the author of this book makes any warranties, expressed or implied regarding the currency, completeness or scientific accuracy or validity of this information nor does it warrant the fitness of the information for any particular purpose. It is intended to provide helpful and informative material on the subjects addressed in the publication. It is sold with the understanding that the publisher and author are not engaged in rendering medical, health, or any other kind of personal professional services in this book. The publisher and author specifically disclaim all responsibility for any liability, loss or risk, personal or otherwise which is incurred as a consequence, directly or indirectly, from the use and application of any of the contents of this book.

Table of Contents

Definitions

1) B.N.B.B.s: Basic Nutritional Building Blocks; concentrated food in tablet, capsule and powder form, including:

Functional-foods designed to elicit a certain physiological response at certain times: *e.g. stabilize blood sugar level, recovery post workout, replace electrolytes.*

Generally speaking, functional–foods are foods which have a higher level of nutrition than non, functional-foods, but more convenient and economical, in nature

The B.N.B.B.s:

- Some sort of protein,

- Multi-vitamin/mineral,

- Good Fats,

- *Pro*-biotics,

- Vitamin B-Complex,

- Vitamin C-Complex,

- Vitamin E-Complex,

- Dietary Fiber and

- Clean drinking water.

2)) *De*-generation: the slow, [often with seemingly sudden onset] process of gradual and preventable breakdown of the essential systems and capabilities of the body.

*When the body doesn't have the B.N.B.B.s and it begins to break down, malfunction, dys-function, manifest syndromes, symptoms, signs, aches, pains, and include fat-gain.

3) *Dis*-ease: the symptoms, mal-functions, dys-functions, syndromes, aches, pains and signs letting us know the process of *de*-generation is well on it's way because the cells need the B.N.B.B.s...*dis*-ease(s), are considered normal and average in much of the medical community to those professionals who do not know about the B.N.B.B.s [through first-hand, personal experience].

*Italics added to [*de*-generative] and [*dis*-ease] as a reminder that they are 'processes' which can be interrupted, rather than 'things we have to live with or have no influence over.

4) S.A.D.C.R.A.P. = Standard American Diet of Continuously & Repetitively Advertised Products:

S.A.D.C.R.A.P. includes but is not limited to:

- Soda pop

- Carbonated beverage

- Candy

- Chips

- Ice cream

- Caffeine

- Alcohol

- Tobacco

Anything with partially-hydrogenated oil, artificial fats, artificial sweetener, artificial coloring, artificial preservatives.

5) Complete Recovery Drink: must be a combination of protein & carbohydrate in a ratio of 2.7 (divide protein grams by carbohydrate grams), re-fuel the body following exercise, training, competition as well as recover from injury, illness, *de*-generation & *dis*-ease.

6) "The Black-Forest of chasing symptoms": refers to the process whereby people taking note of or being diagnosed with a particular health problem, symptom, sign, syndrome and/or *de*-generative *dis*-ease and so forth cover up the underlying symptoms with medication...only to have another symptom appear from the medication itself which in-turn gets covered up with another medication...which in-turn gets covered up by another medication...eventually to find their health so *de*-generated and mixed-up that things seem bleak and hopeless.

7) "Search-and-Consume Mode": when someone has waited too long to eat or drink and they reach for whatever will get them some energy the most quickly...often S.A.D.C.R.A.P...which often leads to a sharp increase in energy followed by a sharp decrease in energy...leading to yet another "search-and-consume-mode"...which cumulatively and ultimately takes one into the black-forest of *de*-generative *dis*-ease.

Every cell of the body [requires] the B.N.B.B.s to maintain, repair and rejuvenate themselves. MOST people are not getting enough B.N.B.B.s for their basic requirements, let alone to burn off excess fat and improve blood chemistry. There are no exceptions. One cannot know if they have enough of them until they do have enough and things that seemed normal simply go away.

Often people attending one of my lectures or reading one of my books will ask, "Yay, but what about my...?" What's the answer?

The B.N.B.B.s!

Yes, some of the cells and systems require other things in addition, but you want to make sure the basics are in place, instead of skipping the basics and substituting other things.

Just like breathing air.

Just like drinking water.

Just like eating food.

Every cell requires them.

One might wonder… *"I have such and such,"* or *"I was diagnosed with this or that…what should I take?"*

Begin with the B.N.B.B.s.

Build upon the B.N.B.B.s.

Every cell requires them.

Done properly, you'll feel so much better and most likely be surprised by all the benefits you experience.

People will be asking you, *"What has changed?…you seem different."*

Introductions

"Until we boldly separate the two concepts of food & nutrition from one another there will always be confusion, debate and resulting subpar nutrition in the body, resulting in subpar body composition (too much fat). The confusion lies in the "one or the other" debate (food or dietary supplements?). Food doesn't necessarily provide consistent enough nutrition and nutrition-density isn't necessarily provided by what we call/think of as food. I've never seen an exception to this." -Sov

For those of us in the fitness industry with enough field experience to reflect upon (from the inside out), the relative strengths and weaknesses of the training system we go through and the information provided to us as health professionals for our certification(s), we realize there is a vast ethical, moral and cognitive dissonance between:

What the consumer of weight-loss marketing information wants to believe is intuitive, in terms of what they need to do to lose 'weight' (what we think is right action):

e.g. "Eat less to lose weight."

What the consumer of weight-loss marketing information wants to believe is intuitive, in terms of what they need to do to burn 'fat' (what we think is right action):

e.g. "As long as I weigh less and get smaller I don't care how it happens."

How much of what is marketed to the consumer of weight-loss marketing information to personal-trainers, fitness trainers and the like pick up and believe to be credible, safe and effective in the long-run (for their clients), and in turn apply or get their clients to "do" as ways of attempting to ratify their own value of service, (promise certain results to gain a client followed, with no way of holding themselves accountable to potential weight-loss goals let alone health improvements for the clients):

e.g. "As long as the client loses weight and gets smaller they won't know if they have done it safely or not and the trainers don't care as long as they get paid."

What is quick, convenient, mediocre in terms of safety, noticeable and yet un-sustainable by the lay-person vs. what is sustainably fast, safe, easy, noticeable as well as clinically measurable as health promoting in the short and long-run for improvement of body composition as well as long-term health:

e.g. The main focus is on the client losing weight in the first six-weeks, regardless whether it is safe and healthy or not.

And finally, the fitness professional's ability to discern between what is weight-loss marketing 'hype' (advertising disguised as information or science to keep a consumer wanting to lose weight as long as possible…keep them buying stuff which promises weight loss, delivers little and makes the body crave things which cause weight gain):

e.g. Even many personal trainers don't know if the information and direction they are providing is safe for their clients, but they don't know how to measure 'safe' let alone hold themselves accountable to ethical practices."

[And its application should therefore be avoided both by consumers and by fitness professionals due to short-term weight-loss in trade for long-term health distortion]:

*e.g. Just because someone loses weight does not mean they got healthier in the process…health should be the first priority, followed by fat-loss…neither are exclusive…*and what is practical, applicable, re-producible science (and its application should not only be adhered to by consumers and health professionals due to short and long-term, sustainable fat-loss but also for clinically measurable and documentable improvements in bio-chemical markers, *e.g. blood pressure, total cholesterol, HDL, LDL, triglyceride levels, blood sugar, insulin sensitivity, etc.* for the top ten *de*-generative *dis*-eases of our time, *e.g. heart dis-ease, diabetes, stroke, obesity, etc.*):

e.g. When one burns fat safely, the chemistry of the body improves and the overall health improves and can be measured by your physician...if the above markers didn't improve, there may be too much emphasis placed on 'weight-loss' first without regard for health.

Which is the metabolically and physiologically sound and yet largely neither marketed nor promoted nor understood by much of the average fitness professional and even less understood by the weight-loss consumer market?

e.g. "I believe relatively few fitness professionals know the difference between weight-loss and fat-loss or the differences in facilitating the two."...for example, a few of the many common and misunderstood concepts regarding weight loss:

- Low fat diets,

- Good vs. bad fat,

- High protein diets,

- Calorie restriction,

- Low carbohydrate diets,

- Attempts at "starving the fat"

- Frequency of meals and snacks,

- Withholding of nutrition-density,

- Quality vs. quantity of fat consumption,

- Exercise without application of nutrition,

- Attempts at weight loss without application of nutrition and

- Attempts at weight loss success through deprivation and the like.

e.g. The things which don't work in the long-run.

These have been shown to produce short-term weight-loss (loss of lean mass along with some body fat), and accompanying disintegration of critical blood-chemistry markers of health *e.g. blood pressure, total cholesterol, HDL, LDL, triglyceride levels, blood sugar, insulin sensitivity, etc.* followed by re-bound affects (re-gaining the weight and more):

e.g. The diet market promotes the concept of the quick-fix without regard for the long-term affects…taking advantage of people's desperation while the practical, applicable, re-producible science:

• Improves bone mass

• Improves lean mass

• Improves blood pressure, total cholesterol, HDL, LDL, triglyceride levels, blood sugar, insulin sensitivity, etc.) and

• Decreases body fat

e.g. Do it correctly and your whole life will improve and get better with time.

routine basis to get what we want. Affirmation make it so your mind pays attention to your environment, in ways which support your primary goals and incentives.

For example: *You want to burn fat,* so you make up a sentence that matches what you want to experience, and you say it out loud to yourself throughout the day, preferably *upon awakening,* prior to sleeping and at one other time. For example:

"I find it easy to follow Results!"

"I am enough."

"Each day, I am increasing my awareness of myself."

"I don't need to weight anymore."

Affirmations work even better when you look yourself in the eyes in front of a mirror, while saying the affirmations and create 'feelings' as though you have already succeeded.

Self-hypnosis:

Self-hypnosis is doing hypnosis with yourself after learning how. You learn to guide yourself into a different, more relaxed and suggestible state of awareness and then you make suggestions to yourself which manifest actions in alignment with your goals. For example, while in trance you say:

"I'm thankful I've burned 45lbs of fat."

"I learned what to do and did it."

"I have relaxed into a lean lifestyle."

"I am enough."

Self-Visualization:

Self-Visualization is simple. All you do is *imagine* yourself as you intend to become…as if you have already achieved that which you desire, while *simultaneously* experiencing the positive emotions associated with your success. If you want to go from a size 12 dress size to a size 8, you *simply imagine* what you look like in a size 8 and flash the image in your mind with *frequency* throughout the day (along with the emotions you'll experience when you have achieved it).

If you want to go from a size 48 waist to a 36 you simply flash that image in your mind throughout the day...the more vivid the experience, the easier it becomes reality.

Most successful people *utilize this simple technique* in one form or another. Golfers, swimmers, track athletes and high-achievers in all walks of life utilize one form or another. Self-Visualization guides the mind toward the intended goal.

Guided Visualization:

Guided Visualization is when a hypnotherapist talks to you, *while you are seated* and *in a relaxed state* of mind that help you *keep your mind and emotions on track* and expecting to achieve your goals. For example:

"You can see yourself having fun, purchasing new clothing, to fit your ideal self."

"You can imagine all the fun you have now."

"You can imagine exactly what you want yourself to look like, before bed and upon awakening."

"You can imagine others commenting how much you have changed."

Clinical Hypnosis:

Clinical Hypnosis is when you are guided into a deeply relaxed, highly suggestible state of mind. New ideas, associations and concepts are introduced as possible ways for you to proceed. For example:

"While you go about your day, you can choose which activities you enjoy the most and which foods make you feel your best."

"You may notice that the new ways of thinking and being are preferable."

"While there is a part of you that remembers the past, another part of you looks forward to the future."

"While people learn some habits as children, adults utilize other habits."

In my experience, all variations *work well* and it is really up to you to *pick and choose* which ones work best *for you. You* and your buddies can *do different* ones and compare your *experiences* when you speak each day.

In my book, *Hypnosis for Good Christians,* I go into greater detail about the most common misconceptions about hypnosis and the role it plays or doesn't play in church, religion, spirituality and so-called 'control' of the mind. Although I'm not an evangelist, it does answer some preconceived notions about hypnosis.

If you are over-fat, you have already relinquished control of part of your mind to food producers, advertisers and other participants of the media. All of which use deficiency of the B.N.B.B.s to maximize their ability to suggest products to your lower/emotional/limbic-brain, so even though you don't want to purchase and eat these things, *you* can't *seem to stop yourself.* That is called a post-hypnotic suggestion. When a person does something, they are told to do, or something they were told would happen. Examples:

"If you eat potatoes, you will grow up to be fat."

"You have big bones, so you can't help but be fat."

"Everyone in our family gets fat, you can't do anything about it."

"When you are in a hurry, you grab a candy bar and feel better."

"The ice cream is so cheap you can't afford not to buy it."

"Ice cream makes you feel good."

"Big butts run in our family."

"You inherited my stomach."

Regarding TV and radio commercials, the more often the message is given, the more likely it is to work. This is called repetition of direct and indirect suggestions. The more repetitive the message the more familiar people become with the product and usually that is the one they use…they think they have a good reason for choosing the product other than seeing it advertised…they tell themselves they aren't hypnotized, all the while carrying out post-hypnotic instructions.

Sitting in front of the television puts the mind in a heightened state of suggestibility. Sometimes it is referred to as the alpha state of consciousness. Just when you get into the program, (an emotionally-open, relaxed state), a commercial comes on and suggests the product they want you to consume. In other words, *the choice you* will *make* is made *before* you even get to the store to shop. It works so well that people buy enough of the suggested products, prices fall and it becomes the most popular product based on price.

…unless, *you put enough of the B.N.B.B.s in your body.*

The B.N.B.B.s help over-ride emotional-based decisions, *interrupt negative hypnosis* so you *make decisions based on your highest held goals and aspirations.*

I found an article on the internet that describes how major retail store chains are using laser-like sound beams to pinpoint individual shoppers to 'encourage' buying with recorded messages. Called hypersonic-sound, the technology is being used in grocery stores in the United States.

The May/June 2004 issue of *Psychology Today* reported that American advertisers spent $12 billion in 2003 targeting the youth market. Part of that money was invested in the 40,000 TV advertisements the average child watches, per year. And that the age at which most children can critically interpret commercials (in other words, prevent the messages from going into their subconscious mind in the form of hypnotic suggestions), is eight years old. For eight years, as children we are [learning before they know they are learning]. Messages about what to eat and how to make choices about food are made for them before they even know it. Their mind-bodies are literally being programmed to become fat.

The type of hypnosis, self-hypnosis, affirmations and guided visualization *I* do *empowers you to make decisions and take action based on your goals and values.* That's exciting to me.

For those of you who don't know me yet, I have no interest in controlling your mind. I do have an interest in empowering you to live the life of your dreams! I love most to see you making choices that are right for you...choices that empower you to live your life to the fullest. I am so busy with my own life that I simply don't give a hoot about controlling others. I offer products and services that help you *get what you want most* and for those that know me best, know that I have never compromised my values, even at the expense of consistent work and housing. If you go to someone else for hypnosis, you have to shop around just like you do with any other health-care provider. Find one that is right for you. Develop and *trust your instincts.* And ask your friends if they know of a good hypnotherapist.

Often people find that when the mind part of the equation is addressed, the *changes* they want *are easier* to maintain until they become healthy, *unconscious habits.* My primary focus is on *de*-hypnotizing people from the fat-producing, effects of television and radio advertising. I shopped around for nine-months, before deciding on a hypnosis school for myself.

Massage:

Massage, body work, Reiki, foot reflexology…they all have their place in assisting you with your fat-loss goals.

In my experience, here's how: When *you are relaxed*, and *I mean really relaxed*, everything is easier. The body is capable of withstanding extreme stress for short periods of time. The higher the stress level, the shorter duration the body is able to cope with it without side effects like cravings, binging and increased body fat.

As long as people are experiencing stress they will find ways to *soothe themselves*. Soothe the nervous system. Soothing may come in the form of a hobby, exercise, support groups and it should always include the B.N.B.B.s. Often, the first thing people do (when stressed) is consume something that changes the chemistry of the mind body very quickly. S.A.D.C.R.A.P. is the most common way. Unfortunately, the emotional-high/effects are short-lived and the end result is that the artificial soothing created more stress and depleted the body of the nutrients and chemicals which help the body heal from the stress.

There are two characteristic-sides to the nervous system. One side helps us cope with emergencies. The other side is total, endorphin-ized bliss. Endorphins are the healing hormones we experience the effects of when we are hypnotized or during massage or bodywork.

Here's the thing. The body is capable of withstanding a lot of stress. Everyone's stress threshold is different and, as of yet, I don't know of a way to know ahead of time how much any one person can handle, over a short period or a long period. Chronic stress kills the body. Accidents and trauma induce stress and often, the body quits working as a result of too much stress in too brief a period.

We are exposed to a lot of stress. Meeting the demands of school work, family, traffic, poor lifestyle habits, terrorism, etc. We live in a higher level of stress on a daily basis than we should have to. What today is considered low to moderate chronic stress should be considered a high level of stress. Because stress exposure is so frequent the body's threshold is raised outside our awareness. We experience stress, the effects on the mind and body and respond to it, without knowing it is stress.

Stress affects everyone differently in the short run and the same in the long run. For many people, in the short run, they gain fat. Excess body fat is a result of stress and creates more stress. For almost everyone, the long-term effect of chronic, low-level stress is early aging and *de-generation* of the body and its systems.

Often, when people are stressed and over fat, they sort of check-out from their body mentally to get some relief. Often this is referred to as *dis-association*. Burning fat is a process of becoming more associated/present to the mind and body, through consuming enough nutrition-density to burn fat.

Being healthy, feeling really good both mentally and physically promotes association to the mind~body. It is a *pleasant experience* and to *experience it fully*, one associates to their body fully, *making fat-loss even easier*.

Many times, people don't feel that great about themselves, so they don't want to be touched. But, massage, energy work, reflexology all have some things in common:

● They 'switch' the body from a stressed state to a *relaxed* state, which makes fat-loss easier and more effective.

● They help you *'associate'* to your body and make healthy choices easier rather than choices based on soothing a stressed mind and body.

● They promote the *release* of *healing hormones and relaxation hormones* to off-set whatever stress you are experiencing in your life.

● You *feel better!*

There are thousands of different forms of massage, bodywork, energy-work and reflexology.

If you don't like to be touched, get hands-off energy-work. If you don't like being un-clothed under a sheet, keep your clothes on. If you only want your feet touched, get reflexology.

Every single body worker has different style even with similar training. Get the kind you like. *Aim* for once a month. If you can afford it, get it once a week. Get *experience* with different styles and have *fun*.

Receiving massage makes it *easier to burn fat!*

These mind body skills and exercises make all the difference in the world. They make *seemingly* laborious tasks *effortless*. Pick the ones you like and *go for it!*

In Chapter Eight I'll cover the steps you want to *do* to *get going!*

Chapter Eight

It's All Up To You

Whether *you* have 15 pounds to lose or 400 pounds or more fat to lose, you will *love this program*. If *you* have never yo-yo dieted, you have yet to *appreciate* all that *Results!* includes. Everything has been taken care of, so *you* don't have to waste a bunch of time thinking about what to do or when to do it. Simply *get* your supplies, get your buddy(ies) and get *going*. This program works when *you work it* and you have the right to *succeed* as much as the right to fail. The results speak for themselves.

Here's your checklist to get you going:

1. Read this book,

2. Contact me for an initial consultation,

3. After that, if you choose, get started with me. My fees are less than most trainers with my level of experience and I'm happy to explain my fees. I get more requests for help than I can personally fulfill, so there's no pressure and I screen who I'll work with based on their initial commitment level, their willingness to take suggestions and their habits of follow-through.

4. If you want to start with me, request and review my suggestions, for you and your eight-week (8 week) journal. Successful fat-loss programs break big goals into 8-week chunks.

5. Find your buddy(ies), you need at least one person who will do the first 8-weeks with you, after reading this book and *Weighting To Wait.*

6. Purchase your whole-foods, functional-foods and B.N.B.B.s,

7. Purchase drink bottles, water bottles, food prep trays, a food scale, body-comp scale, etc., to carry your food and drinks with you to work, etc.,

8. Think about how you will plan your time for activity and to fit in all the foods,

9. Select your start date,

10. Set times to follow up with your buddies, on a daily basis,

11. If your buddies don't follow through, get more buddies.

Let your family, friends and acquaintances know ahead of time that you are starting, so they know you are following a specific health-building, fat-burning journal. By letting them know ahead of time, they are less likely to be offended that you aren't eating their cooking or going out for drinks with them or indulging in the Friday night pizza party or whatever other family and social events are coming up. You're likely to drum-up some extra buddies, too, since they have been looking for something that works!

● Make an appointment with yourselves to exercise and keep that appointment. Burning fat requires keeping commitments to yourself.

● Call or talk to your buddy(ies) after you do these two things.

● If you chose affirmations as your mind skill, do them.

● Check each thing off as you accomplish them.

● Flash across your mind the picture(s) and feelings of you accomplishing your first eight-week fat-loss goal. Create the feelings of accomplishment.

● If need be, prepare ahead for the following day.

● Simply stay on track/keep yourself on track. If you get off track, just get back on track and resume where you left off.

● Think ahead so you can plan ahead.

In Chapter Nine I'll be talking about *The Role Of Detoxifying Yourself For Maximum Fat-loss. See you there!*

Chapter Nine

The Role Of Detoxifying Yourself
For Maximum Fat-loss

You can *speed up* your *fat-burning* process, by *reducing your exposure* to legal toxins by 30%. The less toxins you have going into your body, the easier fat-loss seems, because you feel better.

When I talk about 'legal toxins' I am referring to the onslaught of chemicals we are exposed to on a daily basis, in our *personal* care products like toothpaste, shampoo, conditioner, moisturizers, shaving creams, deodorants, anti-perspirants as well as the artificial colors, flavors, fats and sweeteners in today's low-carb, low-fat fads.

Tens of thousands of chemicals have been introduced into the environment since the 1950's (about 83,000) and few have been tested on an *individual* basis and even fewer have been tested in combination with each other, for their cumulative effects on human health.

Household cleaners, make-up, cosmetics, laundry cleaners and laundry fabric softeners as well as air deodorizing products introduce a chemical concoction, into our personal environment that has never been tested to monitor the results these products have on our *health and welfare*. There are simply too many chemicals and there is no way to know which products any person is going to use at the same time in their home.

The big commercial cosmetic and skin care product companies often test the products on animals, find them to be toxic, irritating to the tissues & disruptive to the hormones yet continue to market and sell the products to the public anyway.

Many, many products now have plastic like components within their ingredients, which remain liquid or soft even when exposed to the air.

These plastic components, and I mean everything from pesticides and yard care products to cosmetics to plastic food containers mimic the female hormones. When we have these products in and around our homes and offices, we are exposing ourselves to things that *promote* what we do not want. When plastic containers are used in the microwave, the plastic is literally forced into the food, resulting in excess fat producing hormones being introduced into the body.

In other words, excessive chemicals promote an increase in the hormones which promote fat-gain, not to mention a general *de*-generative effect on all the systems of the body from the way one thinks, learns and processes information to *sexual and reproductive health and vitality.*

Most experts would *agree* that consuming unnecessary sex-hormones is not a *good* thing. It is kind of *common sense*, wouldn't you say? Yet, since these products are marketed as cleaners and *personal* care products, there are no laws to prevent them from being sold, based on what they are advertised as in the market place. In most cases, products have to be proven to be dangerous, before they will be recalled or pulled from shelves. (Tobacco products are proven dangerous and they're still available!). Since, there is so much money involved, the process takes decades. In the meantime, thousands more chemicals are produced and marketed to those of us who didn't know any better.

The best advice I can give *reduce your exposure to legal toxins by 30%.* You do that by eliminating toxic things in your home and office so at least during these times, you *reduce your exposure to them.* You do this by purchasing only:

• *Earth friendly, people friendly* cleaners and laundry products that have not been tested on animals.

• *Drink purified water.*

• Purchase only cosmetics, skin care and personal care products that are *earth and people friendly*, non-toxic and never tested on animals.

In some cases, full-retail prices for *earth-friendly*, non-toxic products *are* higher than the commercially popular products advertised with *great* frequency, but the way I look at it is that what you pay in price *right now*, you will save in pain and suffering later on. Or, what you think *you save right now* you will pay later in misery and effort to regain your health. You can *shop for deals* the same way you do for everything else.

I began making the switch in my own home in 1993 and I really had no idea *what an improvement* it would make in the way I feel. Before that, I thought there was no difference and that the non-toxic products were simply labeled and marketed as such by the earth-muffins and hippies trying to carve out a niche in a previously developed market. Seriously! That is where I was starting from. I was starting out with a lot of allergies, breathing problems and digestive problems, as well as fatigue from long-term, poor health.

The average, run-of-the-mill yard care products, laundry products, cleaners and personal care products wreak such havoc with the body, but it occurs gradually and over such a time period that we usually do not realize the fatigue, pain, mental fogginess, allergies and inflammation is caused from the very products we buy at the grocery store and proceed to soak our clothing, bedding, towels, washcloths, dishes in or rub on our skin, breathe and dump in our personal environment.

Yet, another form of mass media hypnosis being used negatively for financial gain.

When our personal environment is contaminated with these legal toxins, it is not uncommon to feel like you 'need something to get going' because they literally bog the body and mind down.

One of my *favorite* places to *play* and hang out as a kid was Lake Sammamish, in Redmond and Issaquah Washington. Church picnics, school field trips, watching my uncle race his boat and just hanging-out as a teenager. The water was clean and very warm in the summer. I loved it.

Around 1995 there was a housing explosion on the hills surrounding the lake. All the mass marketed yard care and cleaning products that were being used in the area were running into the lake at a greater rate than the lake could clean itself up. *And this is a lake that has a large slough emptying it* into Lake Washington.

To make a long story short, all those popular 'cleaning' products have phosphates in them which make algae grow much faster than normal. The lake became dead, within a short time and it wasn't until a dog playing in the water died, that action was taken to educate the local residents about *Earth and people* friendly non-toxic cleaners. The lake has begun to *recover* as a *result* and the products still fill the store shelves. They are legal toxins!

In Dr. Paula Baillie Hamilton, MD's book, *The Body Restoration Plan*, she describes how toxins in our environment promote the gaining of excess body-fat. And body-fat produces estrogen which promotes more fat, both in men and women!

Toxins in our food, water, household and personal care products from all-purpose cleaner to skin care and cosmetics contain the chemicals that promote fat by way of the hormones. If you are adamant about succeeding, consider getting the toxic cleaners, personal care, skin care and cosmetics out of your home and you will realize what a difference it makes and how much clearer your thinking becomes.

One of the problems with the low-carb, low-fat rage that is sweeping the nation, is that most of the low-carb products on store shelves is that they are stock full of fake sweeteners, fake fats, artificial flavorings and artificial colorings as well as lack the B.N.B.B.s necessary for life-long fat-loss.

The chemicals in many low-carb products actually promote excess fat gain. They taste great to the person who is deficient of the basic nutritional building blocks (B.N.B.B.s). The chemicals in most low-carb products stimulate the nervous system and confuse the body's feedback system….leading low-carb participants further away from getting to know their body…the essential skill in life-long fat-loss.

Think about it this way: Healthy cells in the body have what they need to burn fat and eliminate it permanently, when the B.N.B.B.s are present. The cells take in what they need, produce energy and rid themselves of waste very efficiently. The concoction of chemicals in low-carb products fill in the empty space within and around the cells with stuff that is of no use in making energy, and at the same time create more waste that needs to be eliminated. In order to eliminate the additional waste, the body has to have more pure water to carry the waste out.

In other words, the body has to 'hold' more water to dilute and get rid of the unnecessary stuff put in the body in an attempt to cope with the low-carb products, just so the cells can do what they would do all *on their own,* when they have the B.N.B.B.s on a daily basis.

You don't have to use low-carb products to *burn fat.*

When the mind and nervous system is sluggish, as a result of chronic toxicity, things seem more difficult. *Aim* to reduce the toxins in your personal environment (your home and office) by 30%. *Replace* the toxic products with non-toxic products. You will *free up* your mental *reserves* for what *you love* most. It will become *easier* to maintain a lean lifestyle.

It is so funny to me when people really *realize* the products they bought at the store are toxic and they decide to convert their home to a 'healthy home'. They still want to use up the last of the toxic stuff because they spent money on it. They may not realize that *poison is no value at any price.* I was the same way *u*ntil I experienced the difference for myself.

I could go on and on here about the horrible tests performed on rabbits and other small animals, while they are held in glass tubes, so they can't squirm away from the stuff being rubbed into their eyes and open sores on their skin. I could talk about the damage being done to the Earth. I could talk about how these companies made chemicals that they didn't know what to do with after the wars, so they call them 'cleaners' and market them to families. But I won't. There are massive organizations dedicated to these causes and you can find them yourself on the internet. This is about you *becoming your ideal self.*

The B.N.B.B.s *detoxify* the body because as the body gets the building blocks it needs every day, it sheds the older cells in favor of *new, properly fed ones* and the body makes *new healthy cells* out of what?….B.N.B.B.s!

The detoxifying formula aids the detoxification by *gently encouraging* the organs to let go unnecessary sludge that builds up a result of toxic products in the home, fake ingredients in diet and low-carb foods, smoking and other S.A.D.C.R.A.P. The fiber literally *scrubs* the body from the inside out scouring the intestines *without harming* them and *absorbing* toxins all along the way *making it easier* to *burn fat faster.*

The protein formula has special ingredients that nature put in there which block the absorption of the fake hormones, I described earlier. This protein speeds the fat-burning process like no other. Most soy proteins on the market are extracted using hexane type solvents which strip the *special* ingredients, leaving the powder inactive and unable to protect you, yet labeled very similarly. You'll learn more about this once you get going.

Partially-hydrogenated oils and fats are one of the most toxic, dangerous and damaging food products available on the market. The lecithin is *good* fat. By taking capsules each day, in combination with the good fats in the B.N.B.B.s your cravings for fatty foods will be eliminated, making it very easy for you to avoid toxifying foods.

As *your body releases the toxins* in favor of *fresh* B.N.B.B.s, the *water* carries the toxins *out of your body.* The *pro*-biotic formula creates a *healthy environment* in the large intestine so unhealthy bacteria do not have a chance to flourish.

When the large intestine is healthy this way, toxins do not have the opportunity to build up and hang around. They pass out of the body quickly. If you want to improve yourself, *look and feel your very best* for the rest of your life and *fit into that clothing* you have your eye on, *reduce your exposure to legal toxins by 30%.* You'll be pleasantly surprised…*I guarantee it.* Chapter Ten includes some extra tips to consider before you get going!

Chapter Ten

Extras

Results! is safe and effective for men, women and teens. Parts of it are fine for children, as well to increase their daily nutrition-density intake.

● Take front and side before photos of yourself holding a newspaper dated the day you begin your program, to show your 'start" body and do the same as you progress, for your 'after' body.

● If you have diabetes, you will still need to monitor your blood sugar levels because sometimes the fruit can make the blood sugar level increase and eating healthy, nutritionally dense products tends to lower blood sugar. The protein does contain some carbs, but since it is combined with the protein it doesn't seem to cause the swings in blood sugar levels like sugary S.A.D.C.R.A.P. If you're currently taking blood sugar control medication, alert your doctor that you are beginning a healthy lifestyle program and your medication may need to be adjusted over the next three months, six months, twelve months as your blood sugar level normalize and the need for the sugar-lowering medications may diminish.

Often people find their *blood sugar becomes more stable* on this program, as it adds into the body chemistry what has been missing.

If you are diabetic and check your blood sugar level regularly, record it daily in your journal, which you'll receive after your consultation and once you have started a training program with me.

If it is not on the check-off list in the journal, don't consume it, unless it is an optional food concentrate. If in doubt, ask me.*

*If you replace one serving of the functional-food with one serving of post-workout recovery drink, you need to mix it with water only and increase your fiber intake by 6 grams, since the post-workout recovery drink does not contain fiber as it's intended to be absorbed quickly.

*You may combine a half-serving of functional-food with a half serving of post-workout recovery drink mixed with water only.

*If you consume the post-workout recovery drink, make a note of it on your journal check list. If you combine a functional-food and post-workout recovery drink, make a note of it on your journal check list. If you consume an extra serving of fiber, due to consuming post-workout recovery drink, make a note of it in your journal check list.

*One serving of functional-foods and one half serving protein powder mixed in water is fine. This half serving of protein powder is in addition to the other two servings of protein.

If you have more than 40 pounds to lose, you have the option of doing the first eight weeks in consecutive order the way they are laid out in the journal or extending each week by one week, doing two weeks of week one, then two weeks of week two, then two weeks of week three, etc.

Your third option is to go through the first eight weeks and then start over with week one and work your way through week eight. Either way, the fat will melt away and you will experience days when you don't seem to be burning any fat followed by days when you awaken five or more pounds lighter. *Results!* is designed to eliminate plateaus or sticking points that 'dieting' and restrictive eating patterns promote, through blood-sugar-stabilization, thereby re-sensitizing your body to the powerful fat-burning affects, of the hormone insulin. So, basically the fluctuations in calories and variations/choices makes your body burn fat faster. We are primarily concerned with how much your body stats change during the eight-week process, even though it is exciting to measure more often. I can speak with you one-on-one to determine how you want to proceed. Calorie-counting is not required, since its all been figured out, within each eight-week journal. If a person has a big goal with a deadline, like a wedding or a beach vacation, then calorie counting can come into play the last couple months of a 6-8month program, but usually calorie-counting and weighing yourself, more than the first of the month is [counter-productive]. Yes, I'm saying weight yourself and check your body composition, the first of each month (that's when it matters). People who weigh themselves more often, without checking body composition do not have as much fat-loss success.

If you have high blood pressure, high cholesterol, high blood sugar, high triglyceride levels, low HDL or high LDL levels, have these levels checked and documented before beginning *Results!*

• Meat is weighed after cooking. All chicken must be without the skin.

• Vegetables are to be measured before cooking. In the first week, all veggies are raw. Measuring after cooking means you got a bigger serving than you should. The four servings are the minimum you need to eat each day.

• Alcohol and recreational drug use is not acceptable on *Results!* as they often cause the blood sugar level to swing and interfere with blood chemistry, as well as rational food choices.

• The eight cups of water listed in the journal are in addition to the water used to mix the functional-foods.

After the first week, additional whole-foods begin getting added in. If any of them make you hungrier, go back to week one and start over. No matter how long you stay on any given week, you proceed in numerical fashion...*never skipping a week* of the journal. But, if you want faster results, you can go back and repeat week one, then pick up with the week you left off on.

If you are on week one for two weeks, you graduate to week two, not three or four, etc. If you stay on week two for two weeks, you graduate to week three...don't skip weeks, regardless how long you stay on each week. There are things built into each week that teach you how food and nutrition affect your health and fat-loss processes. Don't skip anything.

If you go from week three and then back to week one, due to noticing you're still having cravings or hunger, that is related to adding in a food, for the new week, so which de-stabilized the blood sugar/insulin, proceed to week two, after week one.

People who have more than 30 pounds of fat to lose logically would stay on each week for longer since it is unreasonable and stressful to attempt losing that much fat in 8 weeks. Remember, you want consistent, incremental success. When it's working optimally, you may go three or five days without losing any fat, then lose 5% overnight. (For each 1%=2 pounds of fat). This phenomena is related to the body "waiting" to make sure you ae consistently putting in nutrition density. If you skip one part of the nutrition, you simply won't get near the same results.

Everything on the checklist should be consumed every day. This prevents the metabolism from slowing down. The amount of food and supplements actually makes your metabolism speed up. If you change anything you are not doing *Results!* and you have set yourself up for a major regret.

Priorities for the check-off list:

1) Whole-foods, functional-foods, B.N.B.B.s, fiber and water.

2) Minimum of four cups raw vegetables (other than lettuce, greens, parsley & cilantro), per day.

3) The rest of the check-off list.

• Minimum of four servings of raw vegetables every day, with one serving after each cooked meal.

The functional-foods are very, very unique in the way they are processed to preserve the live, enzymatic activity and blood sugar stabilizing effects. No substitutions are allowed. Even though the ingredients and proportions listed on the label may *seem* close or similar to other similarly promoted products, the difference is in the way the products are manufactured and processed affects how well they improve the blood chemistry and blood sugar stabilizing effects. If you substitute a product, you will be very *dis*-appointed and I won't be able to help you.

• Meat is not required, you may substitute with sources listed in the check-off journal.

• Juicing is not allowed as a substitute, as it can raise blood sugar levels and compete with the outcomes outlined herein. Totally different thing.

If you or someone you know has or does experience certain areas of the body that seem stubborn to give up that last bit of fat there are clear reasons why. Although spot-reduction doesn't really work consistently, without extreme exercise habits, nutrition plays the most important role (stabilizing the blood sugar by re-sensitizing the body to insulin, through nutrition-density and low-glycemic processes).

Often the reason behind one stubborn body part has to do with the theory that low-carb fads are supposedly based on. When the body has become resistant to the powerful, fat-burning hormones that promote lean mass, (insulin primarily), it simply can be indicative of high and low fluctuations in blood sugar levels, which corresponds frequently with people who have too much fat being pre-diabetic (insulin-resistance).

Competitive bodybuilders and physique athletes have experimented with these nutrition principles, extensively, since the 1940's to shed that last bit of fat, so their muscles really show off on stage. I am not suggesting you go to the extremes that competitive bodybuilders do, in order to melt those stubborn areas. I am suggesting you eat ultra-carefully. Here's what I mean.

Some foods enhance the fat-burning effect and some help the body store more fat.

In other words, processed-foods de-stabilize the blood sugar and make the body insulin-resistant, so that fat gets stored, but not used for energy (one-way street).

Whole-foods, functional-foods and the B.N.B.B.s combined stabilize the blood sugar and make the body more insulin-sensitive so that the body can once again tap into fat stores for energy* (two-way street).

*(Some research shows that we really don't know where the fat goes, when it leaves the body), but we discuss it as though it gets used for energy, since it is calorically dense. It's simply an easier way to talk about a phenomena, which we don't entirely understand.

The slower energy carbs, also known as "low-glycemic index" carbs like oatmeal and whole grains and multi-source rice combinations, will help the body shed those last pounds of fat. S.A.D.C.R.A.P. or fast-energy foods promote storage of fat.

Anything that really isn't a food, (diet sodas, artificial sweeteners, artificial colors, fake fats, salts, caffeine drinks, tobacco and alcohol) will promote fat storage. Part of the reason is that those kinds of things simply interfere in two primary functions of the basic unit of the body, known as the cells (energy production and detoxification).

The more serious and committed you are, the more strict you will want you daily regime to be. But don't worry, as long as you are consuming enough of the B.N.B.B.s, you won't even miss the fat-producing S.A.D.C.R.A.P. The desire for S.A.D.C.R.A.P. will decrease the first week and be gone within their first four weeks.

• Once you reach you goal/target body-fat composition level, you still eat whatever you want [one day each week] (after you have completed your first eight-weeks). You can repeat the eight-week program, back-to-back, to reach your body composition goal. Meaning, say you have more than 45 pounds to lose, if after 8 weeks you have only lost 45, you can repeat the 8-week process for additional loss. There's nothing unhealthy about the program, it actually improves overall health, so it can be repeated.

[Once you have successfully completed the first eight weeks, the way it's intended, I'll share the advanced fat-burning habits with you.]

• And again, depending on your goals, how serious you are and what your timeline is, your activity level will need to be tailored to your goals so ask for help.

• If you want to burn more fat once you completed the first eight-weeks, simply follow the plan for weeks 5-8 and/or repeat week one.

You learn so much about how each whole-food, functional-food and B.N.B.B. helps your body burn-fat that all you have to do is continue to pay attention to what your body is telling you to do. In general, if you want to continue burning fat, keep doing weeks five through eight. If you experience fatigue or cravings after eating certain foods, go back to week one. The reason being that nutrition density is at its peak in week one, with the lowest amount, of factors which de-stabilize blood sugar and insulin levels. Everyone's starting point of nutrition density in the body and brain is different, but cravings indicate you're still building up a base of nutrition density. When you've reached the amount right for you, cravings are gone. If they come back, you've used up more nutrition density than you have stored, just through the processes of living.

By following *Results! Life-long Fat-loss System©* for eight weeks, you have learned from your body what effects the B.N.B.B.s have on your mind and body as well, and that the real source and function of will-power is of a well-nourished upper-brain through nutrition-density and blood sugar stabilization (re-sensitizing the body to insulin).

You have learned that a desire or craving for S.A.D.C.R.A.P. is a function of your lower brain/limbic brain/emotional brain, not only trying to get you to eat B.N.B.B.s, but also an attempt to keep your blood sugar at a steady level. Now you know that storage of body-fat is a body trying to make sure enough is available when the B.N.B.B.s are deficient.

As you experiment with what most people consider Standard American Fare, you will have clear feedback about how such products affect your health, energy level and mental clarity.

• S.A.D.C.R.A.P. trains the body to build fat.

• With-holding the B.N.B.B.s trains the body to build fat.

• The combination of these two together imbalance the body, resulting in excess body fat (stored energy), yet often a lack of physical and mental energy/motivation (paradox).

By eating some raw fruit or vegetable after each meal, you are introducing live enzymes into your body, which helps the body burn fat, by properly digesting and assimilating whole food (spark plugs of the body).

After finishing your first eight-week cycle, if you gain back five pounds more than your goal weight, resume week one and after week one, continue on weeks five through eight. A secret to staying as lean as you want to, is planning ahead. THINK. If you are going for a drive, going out to dinner with friends, working out-of-town, traveling or whatever, you need to PLAN AHEAD what you will eat before, during and after the event. If you don't plan what you will feed your body, what you feed your body has plans for you. If you Google "food prep", you'll see millions of photos of what and how people who live a lean lifestyle prepare, so they have access to healthy meals and snacks the majority of the time.

Remember, successful people from every walk of life follow a premeditated plan to prevent interruptions in their success momentum...it's about planning ahead.

In my experience, the single most important factor for continued success is eating the B.N.B.B.s every day. Meaning, even if your food isn't the best, put the B.N.B.B.s in to fill in the nutritional gaps.

• Prepare and make it easy for yourself, by having your functional-foods with you at all times.

• By having these on hand, it is easy to take the right actions to get what you want.

• Worst case scenario is being caught hungry without your supplies.

• Check your body composition the first of each month.

• Eat every 2-3 hours. Do not skip meals or snacks. Check everything off as you go. Eat in advance of activity level, instead of waiting to be hungry.

• If you experience low blood sugar or cravings, go back to week one and eliminate fruits, focus on raw vegetables (four to eight cups a day), then after one week proceed to week two and so on.

Add fruit slowly at week two. In other words, notice if you have swings in your blood sugar level. If so, eat veggies in place of fruit. In general, eat one vegetable after every one fruit. Vegetables are more important for getting the results you want. If you can't eat both because you might get full, skip the fruit serving.

Fruit tends to make the blood sugar level rise and fall quicker than vegetables, increasing the likelihood of cravings for S.A.D.C.R.A.P. The veggies eliminate sharp swings in blood sugar level.

One of the most common errors I have witnessed in the nutrition industry is when people are told they have an 'allergy' to certain foods or ingredients, when in reality they have sensitivity due to lack of nutrition-density...if you have a life-threatening allergy, by all means do what your doctor tells you to do.

On the other hand, time and time again people think they are allergic to soy or dairy or something else, but when they consume these functional-foods they don't have any problems. This is due to the way the functional-foods and supplements are processed. Most often, people are actually allergic to the absence of critical enzymes or having more what I refer in my personal experience as a 'deficiency reaction'. In other words, I wasn't really allergic to fiber, I was just having a reaction because I was deficient of the B.N.B.B.s needed to process fiber.

Once I got the B.N.B.B.s into my body, I now eat 50-60 grams of fiber a day, without having to run to the bathroom within minutes, like I did before the B.N.B.B.s

About 94% of all soy products on the market are solvent or alcohol extracted products which are not certified organic nor GMO free, which have the digestive enzymes necessary for proper digestion of the product destroyed in the manufacturing process. Seems stupid, huh!

***All processed meats like bacon, jerky, summer-sausage, sausage, hot dogs, etc. are to be avoided entirely.

Give it a go!

Let's get on with it...*Welcome to Results!*

Pre-training Questionnaire:

Have you had professional nutrition training before? ___Yes ___No

Are you coachable and open to whole-foods nutrition suggestions?
                                                     ___Yes ___No
Would you follow through on my suggestions?   ___Yes ___No

Did you know that your fitness/fat-loss success or lack thereof is about 80%, based on the how well you apply the three parts of nutrition, during/from the first month, of your program?
                                                     ___Yes ___No
Have you had professional B.N.B.B.s training?
                                                     ___Yes ___No

Are you coachable and open to suggestions about which B.N.B.B.s to take, for optimal results? (versus picking a program apart).
                                                     ___Yes ___No

Currently participating in a structured, resistance-training?
                                                     ___Yes ___No
If so, frequency/duration of sessions ?_________________________.

Have you had professional personal training before? ___Yes ___No

Have you had fat-burning cardio-respiratory training before?
                                                     ___Yes ___No

Is it realistic for you to prioritize 3-4 hours [each week] to exercise?
                                                     ___Yes ___No

What is your current bodyfat percentage?_________________________.

How much fat do you want to lose?_________________________.

What has been your biggest challenge(s), in regard to fat-loss?

____.

Pre-training Questionnaire continued:

Are you committed to applying yourself to resistance-training, cardiovascular-training, and the 3 parts of nutrition: (1) Whole-foods, 2) Functional-foods, & 3) The B.N.B.B.s *for at least one year?* (versus a person who starts stuff, but doesn't follow through).

___Yes ___No

With a standard of 12-20 pounds per month, how long could it take you to lose amount of fat, you intend to lose_________________________________.
How many different weight loss programs have you tried, before?

____.

I look for people who have tried a few things that didn't work and who are looking for something that definitely works. Are you the type of person who wants a structured program that tells you exactly what to do throughout the day, so nothing is left to chance?

___Yes ___No

Are you willing to get your B.N.B.B.s squared away, from the beginning of your program?

___Yes ___No

Although you will likely begin to see and feel positive improvements right away, permanent fat-loss requires a lifestyle change. Are you willing to become more fit by committing to a program that definitely works, for at least one year? (versus a short-term quick fix).

___Yes ___No

How long have you been wanting to lose weight?_____________________.

Imagine you have lost all the fat you ever wanted to, have more energy and look better than ever and all that is taken care of. In what way(s) would your life improve, as a result?____.

*You may find it helpful to remove these pages, scan them and email them to me to assist with your complimentary consultation.

Afterword

How I like to work is to do an initial consultation/interview, with people who want my help. During this time, I screen people for particular characteristics, which indicate if this is a good program match for them or not, explain my fees, what is expected and so forth. I am a fairly tough trainer, since clients expect a lot for their money and in turn I expect accountability, so you get your money's worth...but these are some of the reasons my clients get such good results.

How I know a person is serious and ready to be a client and how I take you seriously is when you get your whole-foods, functional-foods and B.N.B.B.s lined up for at least weeks in advance. You have to have your supplies ready in advance and replenish them before you run out. This is sometimes considered a serious program, since there's no days that go by that you aren't sticking to the plan. You're either in/on it or you're not...there's no modified program.

This program is considered Choice/Program #3 in my book *If I Were Her Trainer*, Amazon (2016). For people who want increased strength, cardiovascular-fitness and conditioning, combining this program with a custom-designed resistance training program & fat-burning cardiovascular training is considered Choice/Program #4 in my book *If I Were Her Trainer*.

Once I'm convinced you're serious and a good candidate, and you've purchased a copy of this book I'll email the eight-week journal and shopping list to help make sure you have everything you need to succeed and get the most from each of your eight-week cycles.

Contact me via email and we'll set up a preliminary phone appointment from there. If you choose to hire me as your trainer to get going on this program, I'll be in consistent contact with you, to make sure you're on track and answer your questions, offer morale support and help you succeed on your program.

One of the most commonly asked question by my clients, after a few weeks on this program is, *"Why are my hair, skin and nails looking so much better than they ever have before?"*

I look forward to working with you.

As a licensed health care provider, author, speaker and fitness professional I know from my own experiences what it feels like to want to improve my health, do what I think is right and still not get the kind of results I expected. I am sure you have your own goals and are looking forward to achieving them. I believe you are capable of living the life of your dreams in your healthy, ideal-self body and you will achieve your dreams.

I want you to contact me today and tell me about all the positive benefits you have experienced, as a result of this information!

In my experience, the greatest potential problem is in not educating yourself about it, but in simply doing it.

I cannot wait to hear from you. I especially cannot wait to share your success story with others.

Appendix

For your complimentary consultation, contact the author at the email below or through Facebook Messenger at Sov Valentine:

e-mail:

sovereignmv@gmail.com

My website:

http://sovereign-valentine.mykajabi.com

Sovereign Valentine
CFT, CET, Yft, SSC, SPN, SSF, Cft, GFI, SFI, EMR, CERT, CMCht, Reiki Master

Reasons or Results! Training Systems© 2018

www.ingramcontent.com/pod-product-compliance
Lightning Source LLC
Chambersburg PA
CBHW051756250726
48659CB00001B/440